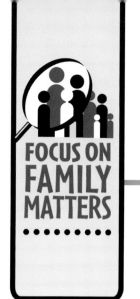

FOCUS ON
FAMILY
MATTERS

Dealing with the
Effects of Rape
and Incest

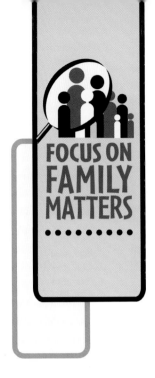

FOCUS ON
FAMILY
MATTERS

Focus on Family Matters

Dealing with the Effects of Rape and Incest

Marvin Rosen, Ph.D.

Chelsea House Publishers

Philadelphia

CHELSEA HOUSE PUBLISHERS

Editor in Chief Sally Cheney
Director of Production Kim Shinners
Creative Manager Takeshi Takahashi
Manufacturing Manager Diann Grasse

Staff for DEALING WITH THE EFFECTS OF RAPE AND INCEST

Associate Editor Bill Conn
Picture Researcher Sarah Bloom
Production Assistant Jaimie Winkler
Series Designer Takeshi Takahashi
Layout 21st Century Publishing and Communications, Inc.

http://www.chelseahouse.com

First Printing

1 3 5 7 9 8 6 4 2

Library of Congress Cataloging-in-Publication Data

Rosen, Marvin.
    Dealing with the effects of rape and incest / Marvin Rosen.
        p. cm. — (Focus on family matters)
    Includes bibliographical references and index.
    Summary: Discusses various traumas inflicted on children and teenagers, particularly
rape and incest, the psychological impact of these traumatic events, and how to deal
with them.
    ISBN 0-7910-6693-2
    1. Rape—Psychological aspects—Juvenile literature. 2. Incest—Psychological
aspects—Juvenile literature. [1. Rape. 2. Incest. 3. Child abuse.] I. Title. II. Series.
RC560.R36 R674 2002
616.85'836—dc21
                                                                        2001008110

Contents

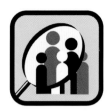

Introduction

Marvin Rosen, Ph.D.
Consulting Editor

B ad things sometimes happen to good people. We've probably all heard that expression. But what happens when the "good people" are teenagers?

Growing up is stressful and difficult to negotiate. Teenagers are struggling to becoming independent, trying to cut ties with their families that they see as restrictive, burdensome, and unfair. Rather than attempting to connect in new ways with their parents, they may withdraw. When bad things do happen, this separation may make the teen feel alone in coping with difficult and stressful issues.

Focus on Family Matters provides teens with practical information about how to cope when bad things happen to them. The series deals foremost with feelings—the emotional pain associated with adversity. Grieving, fear, anger, stress, guilt, and sadness are addressed head on. Teens will gain valuable insight and advice about dealing with their feelings, and for seeking help when they cannot help themselves.

The authors in this series identify some of the more serious problems teens face. In so doing, they make three assumptions: First, teens who find themselves in difficult situations are not at fault and should not blame themselves. Second, teens can overcome difficult situations, but may need help to do so. Third, teens bond with their families, and the strength of this bond influences their ability to handle difficult situations.

These books are also about communication—specifically about the value of communication. None of the problems covered occurs in a vacuum, and none of the situations should be faced by anyone alone. Each either involves a close family member or affects the entire family. Since families teach teens how to trust, relate to others, and solve problems, teens need to bond with families to develop normally and become emotionally whole. Success in dealing with adversity depends not only on the strength of the individual teen, but also upon the resources of the family in providing support, advice, and material assistance. Strong attachment to care givers in a supporting, nurturing, safe family structure is essential to successful coping.

Some teens learn to cope with adversity—they absorb the pain, they adjust, and they go on. But for others, the trauma they experience seems like an insurmountable challenge—they become angry, stressed, and depressed. They may withdraw from friends, they may stop going to school, and their grades may slip. They may draw negative attention to themselves and express their pain and fear by rebelling. Yet, in each case, healing can occur.

The teens who cope well with adversity, who are able to put the past behind them and regain their momentum, are no less sensitive or caring than those who suffer most. Yet there is a difference. Teens who are more resilient to trauma are able to dig deep down into their own resources, to find strength in their families and in their own skills, accomplishments, goals, aspirations, and values. They are able to find reasons for optimism and to feel confidence in their capabilities. This series recognizes the effectiveness of these strategies, and presents problem-solving skills that every teen can use.

Focus on Family Matters is positive, optimistic, and supportive. It gives teens hope and reinforces the power of their own efforts to handle adversity. And most importantly, it shows teens that while they cannot undo the bad things that have happen, they have the power to shape their own futures and flourish as healthy, productive adults.

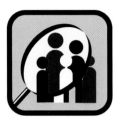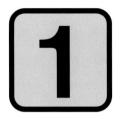

The Hurt
that Lingers

■ Gina had never forgotten. At the teenaged support group, she learned that some children who have been abused seem to bury the hurt for many years before it resurfaces and causes problems. But Gina, who was now fourteen, remembered the hurt all along. She had only been three when the abuse started, but she knew it was wrong even then—he shouldn't have been touching her private parts. Her mother had explained about privacy and what was OK and what was not. But it was her father, and shouldn't he have been bathing her? He had told her not to tell anyone, it was their secret. But when it happened again . . . and again, she did tell her mom. Then things got confusing. Her father left. She didn't see him after that. Maybe she shouldn't have told, maybe it was her fault. NO! She had worked all that out. It wasn't her fault. Her father had a problem. He needed help. He needed to be punished, he might even go to jail. That didn't happen, but Gina went on with her life, living with her mother. She was a good student and had

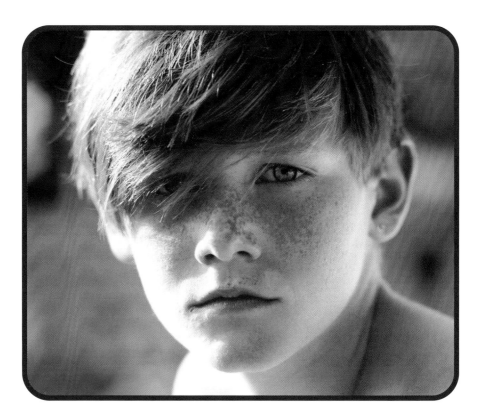

Children expect to have a safe and happy home. When this does not happen, especially in cases of sexual abuse, they lose their ability to trust and often end up with serious emotional and physical problems.

friends. She sometimes became sad that she didn't have a father like other kids did, but there were other advantages. She was an only child and got a lot of attention from her mom. Her Uncle Joe tried to fill in for her absent dad, and he was cool. She'd done all right.

Victims of rape, incest, and abuse suffer for much longer than the time it took for their abuse to be committed. The trauma associated with abuse can be long-lasting, and may affect the victim for years after the event.

However, as this book will show you, there are ways to protect yourself from becoming a victim, and coping skills you can learn to make yourself strong and happy even after you have experienced rape, incest, or abuse.

Bad things happen. We can't control everyone and everything, which is especially true for children. Children are vulnerable and dependent upon parents, relatives, and care givers. We learn to trust at a very young age. We trust that we will be fed when we are hungry, covered when cold, dried when wet. Nurturance and consistency by those who care for us promotes this trust and makes for happy, contented babies and children. But sometimes things go wrong. When our basic needs for warmth and consistency remain unsatisfied, when we are neglected, treated harshly, or abused, our sense of trust is violated. Under these conditions children respond defensively, with suspicion and fear. They learn to be vigilant and on guard. They withdraw and become depressed. They express frustration through **aggression** and defiance. They always appear angry. There is a sense of betrayal that harms relationships and may last a lifetime. Sometimes the betrayal comes later in the form of loss of a parent or guardian, or as an assault—unwarranted, unpredicted, unexpected. When the child has a strong sense of security the assault may be less harmful than if there has already been some emotional vulnerability. Even so, assaults like rape can be devastating, and their effects can be long lasting.

This book addresses such **victimization** of children and adolescents. It covers a wide range of situations that may hurt children, including physical and sexual abuse, as well as incest and rape. In some ways the situations are so diverse you might wonder why they are lumped together. The reason lies not in the physical form of the situations but in their impact, which is remarkably similar. Hopefully, this book will help you better understand why bad things happen and help you cope more effectively when they do. It may prevent the serious emotional consequences of **trauma,** or help you put earlier trauma behind you and find the courage to go on.

Growing up isn't easy

As teenagers and adults, most of us look back on child-hood as a happy, safe, comforting time of our lives. Our parents were there for us, we had few responsibilities, and our needs were satisfied. We felt wanted, loved, and part of a family. Gradually, more was demanded of us. Even though there were now more rules and requirements, especially when we started school, we were cared for and supported at home. We managed to please our parents and teachers and to be generally successful. These challenges and successes made us feel good about ourselves. Adolescence brought new challenges and created stress as we gradually separated from our parents, became more responsible and independent, and looked forward to the freedom of becoming an adult.

This is the image of childhood portrayed in storybooks, television sitcoms, advertising copy, and commercials. For many children and adolescents it is largely accurate, but it is unfortunately not always the case. Sometimes the peacefulness of childhood is violated by trauma, **violence**, and **abuse**. For some, childhood is neither safe nor secure. It is not happy. For others, it is a horror inflicted upon them by people and events at school, and sometimes by those to whom they have looked for trust and affection.

This horror can take many forms. It can occur as abuse by parents or teachers—physical abuse, verbal abuse, and

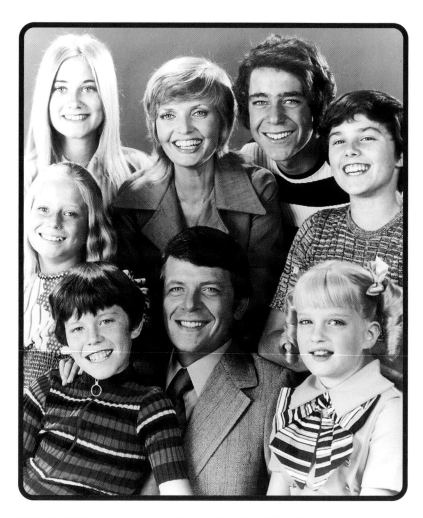

Not all children grow up in happy families like those portrayed on television sitcoms like *The Brady Bunch*. Many children must find the strength to overcome the abuse that destroys this fantasy.

even sexual abuse. It can occur as physical violence against the person, by the continued threat of such violence, or by the experience of being witness to violence. It can occur as **rape**, forced upon a child or adolescent by someone more powerful, more in control. It can occur as **incest**, inflicted by close relative who should be there to help, not harm. These horrors cause emotional damage that becomes part of memory and personality, may last a lifetime, and acts in ways that influence behavior, relationships, and the capacity to trust. This book deals with the impact of rape, incest, violence, and abuse upon children. It points out the devastating effects of such experiences as well as ways of coping with them once they have occurred.

In this book we group several different types of events. Abuse, incest, and rape are not the same. Abuse can occur in many forms—physical, sexual, verbal, and emotional. A person can be the direct target of violence or can be a witness to it. Incest can occur within a family at any time. Some children are the product of an incestuous relationship which can result in serious medical and emotional problems. Sexual abuse of a child by an adult consti-tutes a type of rape. Yet all of these events do share certain similarities. In each, there is a victim and a person who inflicts harm. All of these occurrences can produce a variety of serious emotional and psychiatric problems that are very similar to one another, and each share a need for healing and moving on.

In what ways are rape, incest, and abuse related?

Some definitions

Legal definitions of child abuse vary slightly from state to state. In Pennsylvania, for example, the Child Protective Services Law defines an abused child as any person under the age of 18 who shows evidence of one of the following: non-accidental, serious physical or mental injury, or serious physical **neglect**, or sexual abuse caused by the acts or omissions of a perpetrator.

Abuse refers to traumatic events inflicted by parents, family members, or caregivers to some targeted member of the family. Abuse may be physical and result in injury to the victim. It may be verbal and emotional in the form of demanding and damaging words. Or abuse may be sexual, in the form of rape or incest.

Bruises, welts, burns, fractures, scars and repeated injuries that are not accidental may be signs of physical abuse. Physical abuse may also occur as a physical punishment given as a form of discipline, yet exceeding the bounds of safety and common sense, and done in anger rather than to correct or help. Physical neglect refers to the failure to provide needed medical attention, proper nutrition, and protection from exposure to the elements.

Emotional or mental abuse refers to mistreatment that results in problems such as severe anxiety, depression, withdrawal from friends and activities, and fears for one's safety. These problems must be judged as severe enough to interfere with the child's growth and ability to lead a normal life.

How would you feel if your mom or dad called you names or criticized you all the time? Is this abuse?

Sexual abuse includes touching, rape, **statutory rape**, indecent assault, incest, and pornographic photographing of a child. In these cases, verbal reports by the child and certain behavioral signs are taken as evidence. Rape refers to sexual intercourse with a person when that relationship is not desired or solicited in any way—when the victim has said "no." With a minor below the age of legal consent—18 years old—it is rape even if there was mutual consent but the perpetrator is four or more years older than the minor. Incest refers to sexual behavior between people who are related by blood, whether or not the relationship has involved consent.

Abuse, rape, and incest have long-lasting and devastating effects that persist years after the event, especially if they have occurred consistently over a long period of time. All of these traumas are remarkably similar in their impact.

Some statistics

Social scientists have used various methods to estimate the number of children who are the victims rape, incest, or abuse each year. These figures are difficult to determine for a number of reasons. First, the categories overlap—incest may also involve rape and violence and is classified as abuse. Second, many instances of these crimes go unreported—children may not reveal what is happening to them. Therefore, published figures are usually underestimates of the actual number of victims. Nevertheless, it is important to gather this information to better understand the extent of the problems and their causes, and to plan strategies for the prevention of these occurrences in the future.

Figures published by the *National Clearinghouse on Child Abuse and Neglect* suggest that in 1999 there were 826,000 victims of mistreatment in the United States. This means that almost 12 of every 1,000 children were abused or neglected. The highest percentage of abused or neglected children were in the age range of 0-3 years old. The abuse of females was slightly higher than for males, particularly in cases of sexual abuse. African American children had the highest rates of abuse. It is estimated that 1,100 children died as a result of abuse or neglect in 1999, most under the age of six. Infants comprised 43% of the deaths, and over 80% of their murders were committed by their parents!

Rape is a major crime against women in this country. You may think of rape as some stranger jumping out

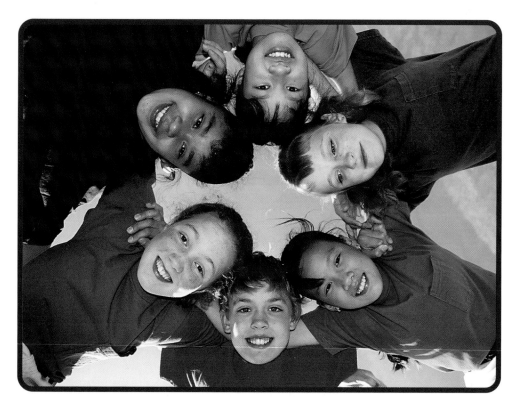

Almost 12 out of every 1,000 children have been abused or neglected, so you may know someone who has been or still is a victim. Dealing with the aftermath of abuse is a difficult process, and one that often requires years of recovery and therapy.

from behind a tree and attacking someone. While this certainly happens, rape is more often committed not by a stranger, but by someone who knows the victim. An all too common rape scenario is that which is committed by someone the victim knows or has dated before the attack. This phenomenon is known as acquaintance or date rape. It has been reported that 92% of adolescent rapes were perpetrated by attackers who knew their

Are you more likely

to be raped by a stranger, or someone you know?

victims. Females 15 to 25 years old represent the majority of the victims. In 1985, a study done on 32 college campuses for *Ms* magazine found that one in eight women had been victims of rape. Yet only 5% of date rapes are actually reported, and even when rapes are reported, the conviction rate is poor. One of every twelve men interviewed admitted to having forced a woman to have sexual intercourse against her will, yet none of them believed themselves to be rapists. Very often the victim does not acknowledge even to herself that she has been raped. No such study has been done at high schools, but it can be assumed that date and acquaintance rapes are not limited to the college campus. The effects of rape, like those of abuse, are long term and can affect the life of both the victim and her family and friends as well.

In Chapter 2, we will explore the causes of child abuse, incest, and rape. The emotional repercussions of such trauma will be discussed in Chapter 3. Chapter 4 presents the legal issues involved in revealing abuse, as well as making false accusations. This chapter will also deal with federal legislation and governmental or private child welfare organizations whose mission is to protect children. Chapter 5 discusses the issue of family secrets and their dangers. Treatment options such as counseling, psychotherapy, and support groups are explored, as are the effectiveness of these strategies in healing emotional scars, regaining control of one's life, becoming empowered, and overcoming one's status as a victim. Chapter 6 takes a broader view and challenges the reader to become informed, suggesting available resources for this purpose.

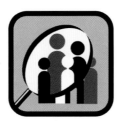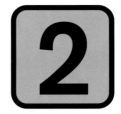

Why Me?

■ Billy wakes up each morning thrashing and crying, "No, dad, no!" He and his sister were abused by his step-dad until his mom found out. She is remarried now, but Billy still lives in a residential treatment center with fifteen other children. Billy sets fires. He became violently aggressive at home and in school. He was sent to a psychiatric hospital but there was no change in his behavior after discharge. Billy is 12 years old.

In a perfect world there would be no abuse. There would be no reason for one person to intrude upon the rights and space and body of another. People's needs would be met and children would be safe. Teens would be allowed to become more independent, enter fearlessly into an adult world, and leave behind childish pursuits. Becoming a healthy and mature adult depends on a childhood free of trauma, want, threat, and fear. Growing children need to feel a sense of security, self-confidence, and respect for

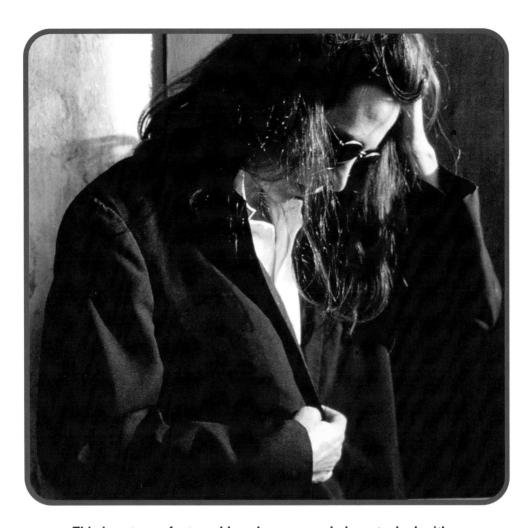

This is not a perfect world, and many people have to deal with issues that may seem insurmountable, such as poverty, racism, abuse, and violence. All of these problems have multiple causes, and must be examined from more than one angle.

others in their homes, schools, neighborhoods, and communities. A peaceful childhood does not always exist, however—bad things do happen, often to good people. Children suffer the loss of loved ones, hunger, illness, disability, and assault. We need not search hard for causes of abuse. They are all around us, and in certain communities they are the norm, not the exception. This chapter looks at the probable causes behind the statistics presented earlier—probable rather than certain because the situation is complex, not simple, and causes are multiple, not singular.

It isn't fair

Who would deny that abuse has roots in social injustice in our country? Significant contributions to abuse have been traced to poverty, **racism**, unemployment, substance abuse, the increased number and availability of guns, inconsistent parenting practices, aggressive role models in families and communities, and the frequent exposure of children to violence on television.

What are some of the factors that lead to abuse and violence in the United States?

About 20% of children live in conditions of poverty. When families are unable to provide proper nutrition, when they lack the basic necessities of living, when they fail to receive proper medical care, when they lack education and vocational skills, when they are discriminated against because of race or ethnicity, and when they live under the constant threat of violence in their neighborhoods, they are at heightened risk of learning to be abusive. People without resources are more likely to give vent to their anger, their frustration, their sense of hopelessness. Children growing up in such circumstances soon learn to enter into a **culture of violence**. This is especially true if they witness domestic violence at home. Furthermore, if they are exposed to murders and assault daily on television, they become less likely to empathize with the pain and suffering of others, and the cycle is repeated from generation to generation. Does this mean that everyone living in poverty must become abusive, that they have no choice, that nothing can be done? Not at all!

How do families contribute?

By now it should be clear that the factors leading to abuse are complex. They include individual, family, and community issues. Family characteristics are the most significant predictors of all kinds of abuse of children. One of the most important of these characteristics has to do with the personality of the parents. Unfortunately, the presence of emotional and mental disturbances in a parent affects his or her ability to raise a child and handle emotions in a healthy manner. For example, anger is a natural reaction to frustrating situations, and is not unhealthy if we recognize the anger and learn appropriate ways of dealing with it. However, anger can be destructive if it is not controlled.

As children we need to learn peaceful ways to resolve problems and disagreements. Psychologists are familiar with people who cannot control their anger, and identify them as having a serious psychiatric condition called **impulse control disorders**. People with these disorders explode when they don't get their own way. Like children, they may have serious temper tantrums, even at an age when they are expected to control themselves. They may be rebellious and defiant. If their behavior becomes so severe that it violates the rights of others, psychologists call the condition a **conduct disorder**. Uncorrected, people with this disorder may engage in abuse and criminal behavior as adults.

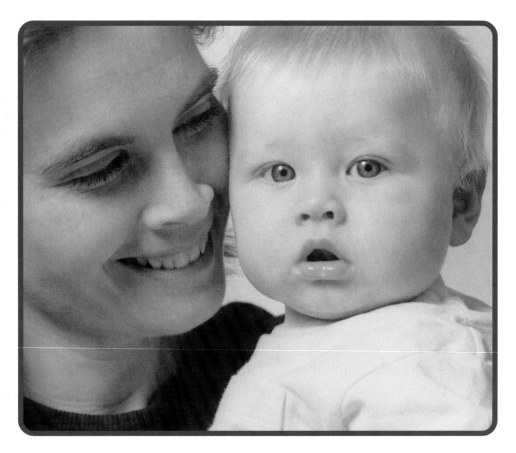

This baby, although young, has already formed an attachment to her mother. If attachment is disrupted, the child may become aggressive and have difficulty raising her own children.

Another significant predictor of child abuse involves a psychological process called **attachment**. Attachment refers to the bond that forms between a baby and his or her mother and father. Attachment is not unique to humans. A newborn duckling attaches to its mother—usually the first object it lays its eyes on. This process can be disrupted. If a newborn calf is taken from its mother immediately after birth then returned after the critical period, the mother rejects the calf. Of course, the process in human beings is far more complex, involving many different factors. Nevertheless, attachment is part of the human condition. It happens with children who are adopted as well as those born naturally to the family. Sometimes it, too, goes wrong.

Even when no serious emotional disturbance exists, the parent may be absent from the home or unavailable to the child during this bonding process. Again, there is no well defined critical period as with animals, but bonding requires the interaction of two people—parent and child. Problems in a marriage and violence in the family may interfere with healthy bonding and even result in child abuse. Parents have different personalities, and may not have the ability to show warmth and emotions, or handle stress, frustration, and anger. These differences can account for differences in their ability to nurture and discipline a child. The parent herself or himself may have experienced abuse as a child, or have been exposed to role models that were violent. On the basis of early experience with its parents, the infant or child learns to expect certain reactions from those around him. These expectations include the child's self-view as someone who is capable of receiving trust, warmth, caring, and consistency from others.

The way a person reacts to certain situations as an adult is influenced by their experiences as a child. Psychologists who have studied a mother's interaction with her baby found that children whose mothers responded quickly to their crying were more affectionate towards her.

How would you feel

if you didn't have a close relationship with your mother?

Children whose mothers were insensitive to their cries

later avoided their mother and showed little prefer-
ence for her over a stranger. These children were also
more aggressive towards their mother at home. These
observations show that the attachment, or bonding,
that takes place between a mother and child in infancy
is very important to how someone reacts to situations
later in life.

Problems in attachment that start in infancy usually
continue through adulthood. Adults who have had
secure attachments as children are more comfortable in
expressing emotions, more self-confident, and more
trusting. Psychologists believe that adults with insecure
attachments are more fearful, shy, and less competent in
raising their own children. Their failure to form secure
attachments with their mothers as infants may result in
a greater chance that they will commit child abuse. This
abuse can take many forms such as open rejection,
greater distance from the child, more severe punishment, or the absence of consistency with alternating
acceptance and rejection. The infant is sensitive to the
discomfort of the parent and learns to mimic the
emotional state of the parent. Rejection leaves the child
feeling unloved and unwanted. This is particularly true
if the parent is being physically or sexually abusive. The
child learns to avoid the parents or concludes that
bonding is not important.

There is also a greater chance of incest between
siblings when parents maintain a distance and are
inaccessible to their children. Children growing up with
parents who themselves have **attachment disorders** may
be more likely to use others, even their own children, to
satisfy their needs when they are adults. Women who
were sexually abused as children are more likely than
others to have daughters who become sexually abused.

Those who have been victims, and who feel alone and distrusting, may later abuse others without understanding the pain they are causing their victims. This possibility would account for the transmission of abuse from one generation to the next.

As you will see in the next chapter, the effects of violence are similar to those of abuse. The transmission of violent tendencies from one generation to the next is also common—a small percentage of families commit a great amount of violence. Some children learn to be violent. Others seem to have a built-in resilience to violence, even though they have been exposed to it. Violent behavior is viewed as the result of inadequate learning of socially acceptable problem-solving skills. Children are rewarded for violent behaviors rather than for emotional control. Research suggests that there is a difference between those children who become violent early and those who start late. When violent behavior starts early in childhood, it is believed that parents are using harsh methods of punishment to deal with bad behavior. These parents correct their children with anger, they fail to set consistent limits, and they use force. They do not teach children socially appropriate behavior. Children learn early that violent behavior pays off. These patterns are associated with serious violent behavior in later years.

Children who do not become violent until later in childhood usually learn these behaviors from influences outside the home, such as neighborhood gangs. Adolescence is typically a time of rebellion against parents. Outrageous behaviors and styles of dress appear to be designed to irritate parents and other authority figures and to gain acceptance of peers. The desire to be "one of the gang" temporarily replaces the need to do what a parent expects. Teens may identify with groups whom they see as oppressed or disadvantaged. Involvement with drugs is one way to express rebellion. The gang may substitute for the family so that the adolescent develops a sense of loyalty that is more powerful than society's norms in influencing behavior. These tendencies, of course, become more extreme when there are already attachment disorders or poor **impulse control**.

Not by a stranger

The problem of rape overlaps that of abuse and violence and many of the same causes are involved. We focus separately here on **acquaintance** or **date rape**, which is a problem primarily for adolescent girls, especially those between the ages of 15 and 25. Only 5% of date or acquaintance rapes are ever reported. Rape is a complicated act resulting from problems in communication differences in the way boys and girls are socialized in our culture. Date rape can occur even when other people are relatively nearby—such as upstairs at a fraternity house when others are partying a floor below. When girls enter a car or apartment alone with a boy they are vulnerable. One frequent cause of date rape is the use of alcohol and other drugs: a boy may become sexually aggressive or take advantage of a girl when either or both of them have been drinking or using drugs.

What would you do
if your boyfriend pressured you to have sex when you didn't want to?

While competitive and aggressive behavior are acceptable in some aspects of life, such as in school and sports, they are never acceptable in an intimate relationship. In fact, it is

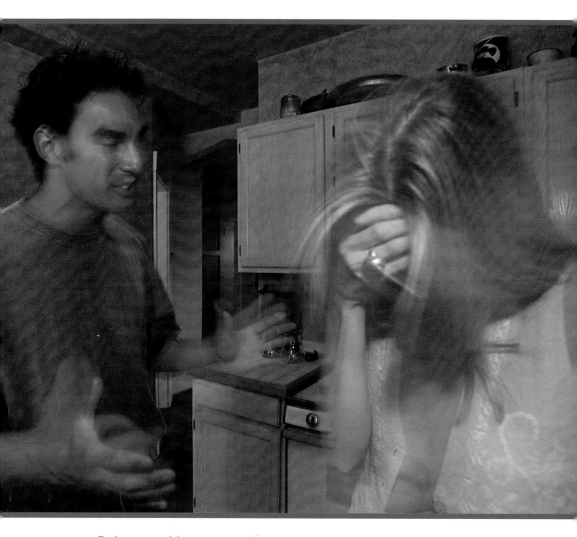

Being raped by an acquaintance or friend is statistically more likely than being raped by a stranger, and carries with it numerous emotional complications. Often, victims of rape feel too confused or ashamed of their situation to report the rape—only about 5% of date or acquaintance rapes are ever reported.

this type of behavior that often leads to date rape. When someone says "no" to sex, it is important to listen to and accept that decision. It should not be misinterpreted as playing hard to get or teasing. Forcing anyone to have sex against their will is an act of violence; no matter how this act is interpreted by the perpetrator, it is rape, and creates a victim who will have to cope with a lifetime of emotional repercussions.

Who would do such a thing?

Other causes of abuse are the characteristics of the perpetrator. People who sexually abuse children vary widely in age, occupation, income level, marital status, and ethnic group. A large percentage of sexual abusers are juveniles themselves. A significant portion of adult sexual offenders began molesting children when they too were juveniles. Ninety percent of sexual offenders are male. Many were themselves victims of sexual abuse. Adults who sexually abuse children relate better emotionally to children and become sexually aroused by them. They are unskilled in meeting their needs with adults. They also have poor impulse control, which is often aggravated by alcohol or drug abuse.

What about TV?

Finally, we cannot ignore some experts' opinions that we have created a culture of violence in this country that perpetuates abuse. The rate of violence is escalating in our large cities. Yet the problem is not restricted to the inner-city "war zones." It is not limited to any one community or group. All children are affected by the violence that pervades our society. It is perpetuated by the media, particularly television and films, and a broadcasting industry that has been deregulated. Children who are frequent viewers of violent TV series may be less likely to show empathy towards the pain and suffering of others. Even children's cartoons contribute to this situation, and many commercial toys seem to promote violent behavior. No child in America today is exempt from such exposure.

Effective action in preventing abuse is therefore no simple matter. To solve these problems, we must also solve many of the problems society as a whole faces.

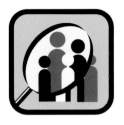 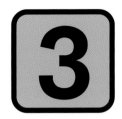

Coping with Your Emotions

■ When Sarah was 10 and her brother was 12, their parents started a family business that took all of their time and attention. They felt abandoned by their parents and turned to each other for comfort. The relationship became sexual. They both knew it was wrong but couldn't stop, and the incest continued for about a year. Eventually, Sarah revealed what was going on to their parents, who put an end to it.

Sarah has carried a sense of guilt ever since and has compensated by trying to be a good daughter. She still feels anger towards her parents for not providing adequate supervision and towards her brother for abusing her, but her real issue is one of trust and betrayal. She has trouble forming relationships and blames this on having been sexually abused.

The effects of trauma and abuse are variable. Some victims suffer no obvious ill effects. Some have mild symptoms. Some suffer serious and long-lasting psychiatric disorders.

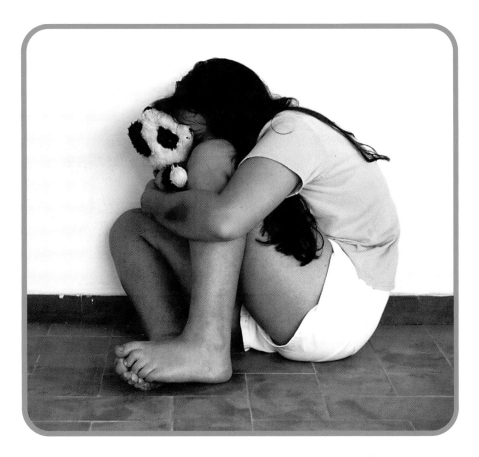

Everyone reacts differently to sexual abuse. The intensity of the emotions one feels, the psychiatric disorders that result, and the behaviors that abuse generates all vary between different victims of different types of abuse.

This variability is not surprising since trauma varies in intensity and frequency of occurrence. It could be a man exposing himself to you in a park. It could be a kidnapping and rape at knife point. It could involve many forms of mistreatment over a long period of time in a chaotic family situation. Furthermore, children differ in their vulnerability or resistance to abuse depending on the amount of support they receive.

This chapter describes common emotional reactions to

abuse, rape, and incest. If you have been abused you may be experiencing all of these feelings or just some of them. Only you know how intensely you feel. Be aware that you are not alone in having these emotions. Other people who have had similar traumatic experiences feel the same way. Also recognize that you are not helpless and can do something about it.

On being a victim

The overriding outcome of trauma is the conviction that you are a victim—that you have been victimized in the past, and that you will always be a victim. The past cannot be changed, but the future is within your power to change. Being a victim is a state of mind. It involves a psychology that is learned and can be unlearned. This chapter asks you to challenge

What can you do

to make sure you won't be a victim in the future if you were victimized in the past?

thoughts that go through your mind on a regular basis. These thoughts are often difficult to change because they have been around so long that they feel natural. These thoughts are linked to emotions. If the thoughts are negative, the feelings they generate will be negative as well. They will consist of guilt, shame, fear, helplessness, and feelings of inadequacy. But they are your thoughts, you are in control. If you change the thoughts from negative to positive, you can change your feelings in the same way.

One of the most damaging emotional problems resulting from trauma is an inability to trust. The inability to trust will be especially severe if the perpetrator of the trauma has been a parent. Our development is closely determined by learning a sense of security from

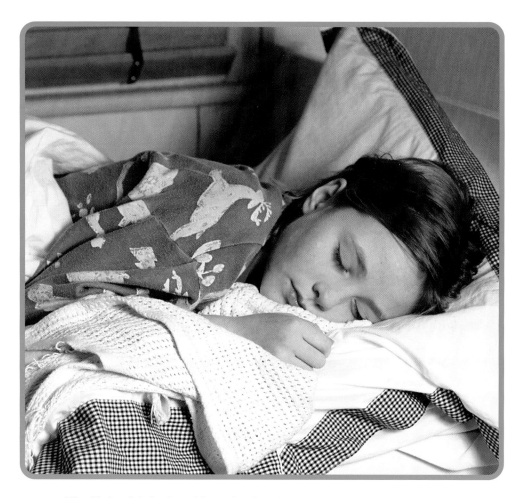

The little girl depicted here is sleeping soundly, but victims of child abuse often lose this ability. Nightmares, bedwetting, and insomnia may occur in abused children, all of which are the consequences of the terrible violation of trust that has been perpetrated on them.

our parents or guardians right from birth. When a child learns that it is dangerous to trust a parent, then why should anyone else be trusted? Inability to trust will make it unlikely that the individual will be able to form close and lasting relationships.

Fearfulness follows from trauma. When you have been

assaulted, it is a natural consequence that you will become wary. You are sensitized to further attack. Caution, heightened vigilance, and a sense of danger become second nature. These are all forms of anxiety, and may express themselves as bad dreams or flashbacks. You are never at ease. You feel that you must never let down your guard. Relaxation is difficult.

It is natural to feel angry after you have been abused, physically harmed, or frightened. Some victims harbor an unrelenting sense of resentment. They can't seem to let go of their anger. Anger can be a complex emotion. We learn as children to control our anger, our anti-social feelings, and to turn the other cheek. We are punished as children when our anger gains the upper hand and we erupt in temper tantrums and become aggressive or destructive. Anger may be buried so deeply we are no longer aware of our feelings. However, repressed anger festers and appears in many subtle ways. We may act in a passive manner, and others may recognize how negative we are being. When confronted, we are surprised and deny any negative intent.

People who feel victimized, threatened, fearful, distrusting, and angry are not happy. They don't feel good about themselves. They may reach the conclusion that they were really at fault. They may think that they did or said something that brought about the trauma, abuse, or rape—that they really wanted it to happen. It is a common occurrence that people blame the victim; it is equally common for the victim to blame herself. Whatever bad happened to them, they feel that they must have deserved it. If you attack yourself in your thoughts, if you turn your anger inward, you will become depressed.

Is it your fault

if you become the victim of rape or incest?

How serious is it?

Physical and sexual abuse can be devastating to the mental health of children. Psychiatric symptoms may include aggressiveness, anxiety and fear, depression and suicidal tendencies, sexual problems, disorders in thinking and concentration, and drug use. Children who have been abused become highly sensitive to further abuse. There may be bed wetting and difficulties falling asleep. They may withdraw from other children. Children often develop a sense of helplessness and lack of control over their lives. Sometimes there is a splitting off of memories so that traumatic experiences, including the abuse, are recalled only in **flashbacks**, nightmares, and night terrors. We call this condition **post-traumatic stress disorder**, or PTSD. Children who blame themselves for the abuse may live with guilt and shame in ways that affect their ability to cope with many problems.

I saw it happen

There are three types of reactions associated with being exposed to or witnessing violence: the development of aggressive behavior, post-traumatic stress disorder, and problems with forming relationships. The similarity to reactions of abuse, rape, and incest is obvious: children may develop anxiety, sleep disturbances, flashbacks and intrusive thoughts, avoidance reactions, and a numbing of emotional reactions to aggressive behavior. It is thought that exposure to violence in early childhood makes it difficult to express feelings or even to tell the difference between emotional states in other people. The younger the child is, the greater the impact of violence will be—children who experience violence before the age of eleven are three times as likely to develop psychiatric symptoms than those who experience such trauma as teens. They have more difficulty focusing on

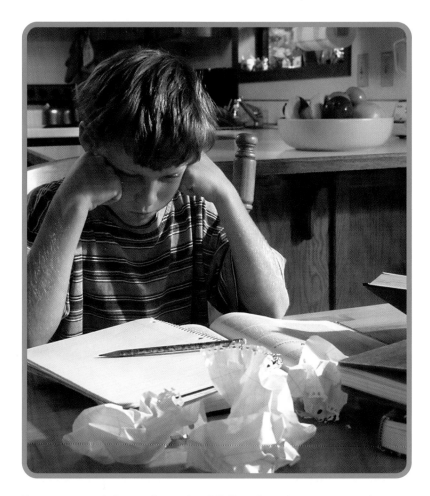

Exposure to violence in early childhood can cause a number of psychological problems, such as an increased propensity to violence, attention disorders, withdrawn personalities, and difficulties forming close relationships. The good news is that up to 80% of children who experience violence can recover without serious long-term emotional consequences.

school work and enjoying many of the activities that most of their peers enjoy.

Children are not the only ones to suffer from climates of violence in the community; parents do as well. Parents who live in such communities frequently describe a sense of frustration and helplessness, and they may communicate these feelings to their children. They recognize that schools, churches, community centers, and even law enforcement agencies are powerless to provide their families with a safe environment. Exposure to violence may interfere with the normal developmental process of the child—a process dependent upon the interactions of parents and children in safe environments. Parents may become overprotective, afraid to let their children out of sight, rather than encouraging increased independence. Professionals working with families in such communities need to acknowledge the reality of such conditions. Under these circumstances, it is understandable that parents will be controlling and protective.

How does living in a violent community affect the way you handle your emotions?

However, exposure to violence does not affect everyone in the same way. It has been estimated that as many as 80% of all children exposed to violence are not seriously damaged emotionally. It is likely that a child's early experience and individual characteristics may serve to protect him or her from the negative effects of traumatic experiences. One significant protective factor is the presence of at least one parent or significant adult who can cope with dangerous environments and develop a warm, supportive relationship with the child. Parents who teach children to deal constructively with problems help build a child's resilience to trauma.

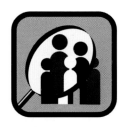 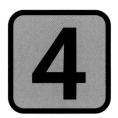

Children Have Rights, Too

■ A young and not very well-trained case worker was assigned to a foster family caring for a three year old girl. Although there was little evidence, the worker "had a feeling" that the child was being sexually abused. She asked an older male foster child to hold the little girl while she lowered her underpants to search for evidence of sexual bruising.

Both children's rights were violated by this worker.

You did not always have rights. In the 18th century, when the United States was a new nation, children were viewed as miniature and imperfect adults. Children were to be "seen and not heard." The father was head of the household and the family, and the Church was the ultimate authority. Children were the sole responsibility of their parents, who had the job of administering discipline. Disobedient children were "bound out" to the local blacksmith or carpenter as apprentices and expected to earn their keep. They were viewed as needing to

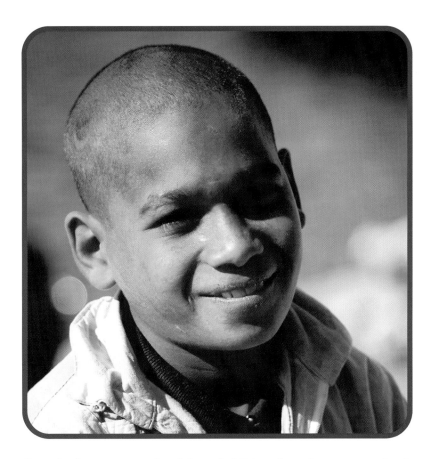

Over the last century, the rights of children have been recognized and enforced by law. If parents are not capable of providing their children with basic necessities, the federal government can intervene to provide help or remove the child from a dangerous situation.

be "saved." By the mid-19th century, the proper education and health of children was emphasized, and schools began to accept responsibility for teaching socially appropriate behaviors by the 20th century. The 20th century also brought a greater understanding of the environmental and cultural influences shaping children, and child psychology became popular as parents sought advice on the best way of raising their children.

The era from 1920 to 1940 was one of great concern

about social welfare. Children were seen to be at risk and were protected by new laws against exploitation at their jobs. The **civil rights movement** that began in the 1950s led to increased demands by all groups for full benefits as citizens. During the presidencies of John F. Kennedy and Lyndon B. Johnson, there was a growing optimism that new technology

How have your rights as a child changed throughout the history of the United States?

and improvement of environments would eventually solve all social problems. Programs such as Headstart and the mainstreaming of handicapped children are two examples of the changes that were taking place then and are continuing today. All of these changes indicate that the rights of children were being recognized.

During the past forty years there has been a dramatic change in the way society recognizes human rights. This change has affected minorities, women, the handicapped, and disadvantaged people in schools, the workplace, and the community. Now, as never before, there is an awareness of the inequities that existed before. Massive efforts were begun by courts and legislative bodies to correct past injustices, including those injustices suffered be children.

In 1979, the Polish government proposed a policy dealing with children's rights, called a convention, which has since been ratified by many countries all over the world. The preamble to this convention states that parents are important for the development and well-being of the child, who needs to grow up in a loving and caring family environment in order to develop its highest potential. The articles of the convention specify the necessities to survival and development, including food, housing, clothing, medical care, education, care, and play.

Countries that cannot afford to provide such guarantees are eligible for technical assistance. Protection of children specifically refers to protection from separation from family, and protection from all kinds of exploitation, cruelty, and violence. Special protection is required for handicapped children, children from minority groups, and children without parents. Children are entitled to express their views with regard to decisions affecting their lives. This does not mean that children have the right to make all decisions; age and level of maturity must be taking into account. The child's right to a private life was also discussed by the convention.

What would you do if you disagreed with a decision that your parents made about your life?

This convention was modified and improved upon over a 10-year period, and in 1989 was adopted as an international human rights treaty by UNICEF. The **Convention of the Human Rights of the Child** is far more detailed and elaborate than the 1979 convention, and affirms funda-mental human dignity and the family's role in children's lives, and seeks respect for children as long as it is not at the expense of another's human rights. The convention reflects the consensus of opinion of most nations and is the most widely accepted human rights treaty ever written. It has been ratified by 191 countries. While the United States has indicated its intention to ratify, it unfortunately remains the only industrialized nation and one of only two United Nations members who have failed to do so.

However, the United States did begin to pass federal legislation in 1974 that identified multiple injuries and bone fractions in children as **battered child syndrome**. These laws support state and local efforts to prevent child abuse and neglect and require mandatory reporting of

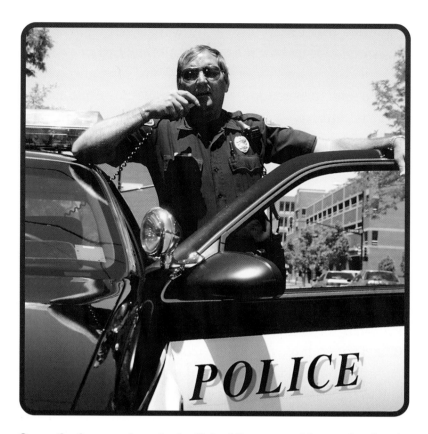

Currently, there are laws in the United States requiring professionals that work with children to report suspicions of abuse to the proper authorities for investigation. Allegations of abuse are very serious – they put into motion a complicated process of inquiry and examination – and should not be made lightly or without serious consideration.

suspicious injuries. President Clinton signed the National Child Protection Act in 1993.

You must be heard

It is essential that families, schools, courts, and legislators recognize the rights of children. But you need to be aware of your rights as well. When you recognize that your rights are being violated, you need to seek help. It is the responsibility of any person who works with children and is aware of abuse to reveal that abuse to child welfare authorities. "Hotlines" exist for this purpose. When an allegation of abuse has been made, the child welfare agency must conduct and investigation immediately. Trained social workers conduct these investigations. Failure to report a known or suspected abuse can result in a serious fine and a jail sentence for the person who does not report the abuse.

Sometimes a false allegation is made—there are over three million child abuse allegations reported in the United States each year, but only one million can be substantiated. This means that over two million allegations cannot be proven. These occur for many reasons—sometimes honest mistakes are made and sometimes it is an attempt at revenge against the person being accused, such as during a bitter divorce. It is not possible to stop false allegations, and this is the only price society must pay for protecting its children. Making an allegation of abuse is very serious, and there have been instances when an innocent person has been embarrassed or harassed. The child must also be questioned and often there will be a physical examination to find evidence. A person's privacy may be invaded, but the suspected abuse must be reported. The need to protect children outweighs the right to privacy.

All people working with children are required by law to report abuse or suspected abuse when they learn about it. Even the **privileged communication law** between a psychiatrist or psychologist and a patient does not hold in cases of child abuse. Everyone is morally responsible to report and interfere with abuse.

> # Would you expect
> a psychologist or teacher to report abuse, even if you asked them to keep it a secret?

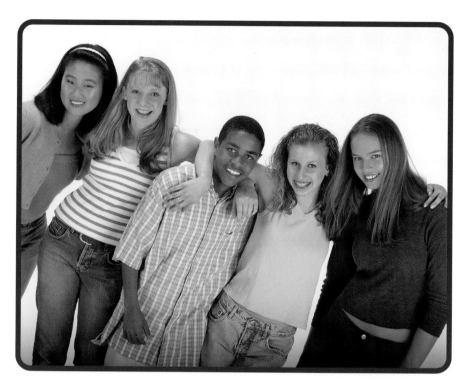

The message of all of the legislation and mandatory reporting laws for child abuse is that children are people, too. As such, they deserve to be happy, safe, and healthy. They have the right to speak out about abuse in their lives in the hopes that it can be stopped, and they can start to recover.

What does all this change mean for you? It means you have the right to speak out when you have been mistreated. It means there should be no victims. It empowers you to be strong, to know what is right, and to protect yourself from injustice. Family secrets should not be allowed to perpetuate the hurtful acts of the cruel, uncaring, or mentally ill people who abuse children. It entitles you to look deeply at yourself and like what you see, no matter what has happened to you. It challenges you to move forward and become the very best person you can be, without regrets. It tells you not to forget what happened, but also not to let it take over your life. It encourages you to be an advocate for others who have been victimized. It means that you need to report the abuse of others. If a friend confided in you that she is being raped or physically abused, what would you do? Suppose she swore you to secrecy? Life sometimes presents tough decisions. The highest priority is to protect children from harm—to keep them safe. When someone is not safe and you are in a position to sound the alarm, promises may need to be broken.

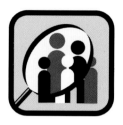 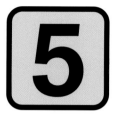

Healing

Martha sat in the therapist's office, chattering happily about her upcoming school prom. This was her third weekly therapy hour. Martha had been referred for flashbacks, a vivid reliving of earlier traumatic experiences that appear real to the individual experiencing them. She had a history of sexual abuse. She was only four when her father started abusing her. Many children seem to forget these experiences for many years, but Martha never forgot. At age 16 she was a good student and popular in school. But she was angry and resentful at what her father had done to her.

Although Martha found it difficult to talk about the abuse with her mother, she opened up easily in her therapy sessions. She told her therapist that it was a relief to talk to someone she trusted about her feelings, to let go of the anger and sadness she had bottled up inside of her.

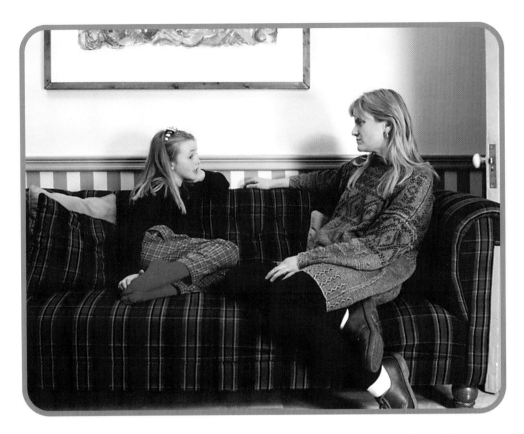

An important way for children to stop abuse or correct harm is to talk about it with a trusted family member or adult. Open communication can also help a child work through a personal issue.

In families that function well people talk to each other—not just basics like "pass the milk" or "I need lunch money," but significant talk about feelings, ideas, needs, hopes, and wishes. This doesn't always happen after a traumatic event, when it is most critical that the channels of communication remain open.

Growing pains

Adolescence is a time of increased turmoil and stress. Body changes occur rapidly, creating imbalances in personality as well. Teens experience extremes of emotions which can be confusing to them as well as to those who live with them. Feelings of inferiority and insecurity are not uncommon during these adolescent years. You worry about bodily changes, and whether or not they are normal and working right. There is a heightened need to master challenges, to be competent, to be independent.

This need for independence results in a distancing from parents and often a rebellion against the rules and values parents have instilled in you. This condition is temporary, but may cause friction between you and your parents for several years. One repercussion is a breakdown in communication with your parents— a lapse that can be damaging if, during these rebellious times, you suffer trauma and no longer view your parents as your primary support. The trauma is kept secret sometimes between the perpetrator and the victim. Without realizing it, parents may respond in ways that increases the distance from their teenage child.

Most teens today enjoy a degree of freedom unequaled by previous generations of adolescents. And with the new freedom comes increased responsibility, challenges, and stress. Those who have studied teens report that they live a life of their own, so that most adults do not have a clue about who you really are or what pressures you face in your daily life.

Journalist and writer Patricia Hersch decided to find out about teen life for herself. She selected eight teens in the town of Reston, Virginia. These teens represented a whole range of adolescents from seventh to twelfth grade. Hersch studied them intensively for a period of five years. She not only interviewed them repeatedly, but also got to know them as friends. She went to school with them, entered into their lives, observed their social relationships, and followed their overall developments as persons. She tried to understand them from their own perspective, in their families, at school, and in their community.

How would you really feel if your parents weren't involved in your life and didn't make you follow any rules?

Hersch concluded that teenagers are "a tribe apart." Society, she says, has left you to make their own decisions, to determine your own fate. You attend school, even get good grades. You participate in sports, get jobs, and graduate. Yet these accomplishments, and your success in avoiding pregnancy and drug addition, does not mean that you are happy or out of trouble. Hersch sounds an alarm to all parents to reconnect with their teenage children. "Every adolescent needs a mentor, not just the 'deprived' kids of the inner city." Kids need adults to listen to them and serve as role models. Grown-ups, by their presence, convey a sense of safety and control. "The turbulence of adolescence today comes not so much from rebellion as from a loss of communication between adults and kids and from the lack of realistic, honest understanding of what the kids' world really looks like."

If Hersch's conclusions are accurate, the teen who has experienced or is experiencing rape, violence, or abuse may be reluctant to talk with their parents about it. Fear, shame, and guilt prevent revealing, which is the start of healing. Family secrets will prevail.

In Chapter 2 you learned of some of the repercussions of abuse and violence. This chapter suggests what victims can do to heal their scars. Be aware that the effects of trauma can be serious and long lasting. Advice is cheap. In no way does this book downplay or make light of the pain people feel. It is written with respect for the reader who may have suffered from the experiences. We recognize that overcoming trauma is difficult. That there are no simple solutions.

The first step

First, your must reveal what has happened to you. Keeping secrets about rape, incest, and abuse makes things worse. This doesn't mean that you need to reveal it to the entire world—it is sensitive information and you must be selective about whom you tell. But keeping it to yourself means that you have to handle it yourself. There is power in unloading something that burdens and pains you to someone who will be sympathetic and can find you the appropriate support. Admitting that it happened, first to yourself and then to significant people in your life, takes courage but is the first step toward healing. When revealing also means exposing someone who is close to you as the perpetrator of the trauma, it is very difficult. It will mean an investigation and fact finding by appropriate child welfare personnel. It may mean court testimony, and it may mean someone will go to jail. Even if this is so, it is once again essential that you don't blame yourself. By revealing, you are doing what is right, and what the law requires you to do.

> **What would you do**
>
> if the person who raped or abused you was a relative or close family friend?

Therapy works

If your emotions are so intense that they interfere with your school and social relationships, help is available. Psychotherapists and counselors are available in your

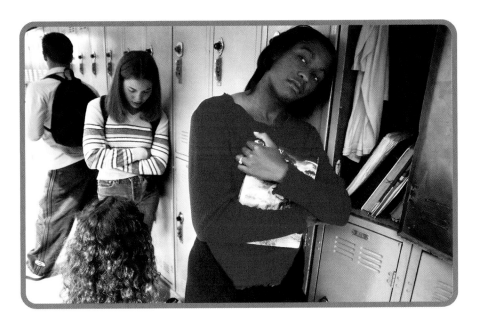

Adolescence is a difficult time, even for teens that are not being abused. There are social pressures and physical changes in adolescents that can be overwhelming – dealing with them in a healthy manner may sometimes seem impossible, but it is not with the proper resources, such as family, friends, school counselors, and mentors.

community to help with the pain. They are trained to help you challenge your damaging thoughts and to teach you survival skills. There are experienced in helping teens deal with trauma.

Not all therapy or thera-pists are the same. There are different schools of thought and different approaches to therapy. Psychologists who have studied the effective-ness of psychotherapy with

Would you be willing

to talk to a therapist or counselor if your emotions were more than you could handle on your own?

sexually abused children found that it works best under certain conditions. When there is a high degree

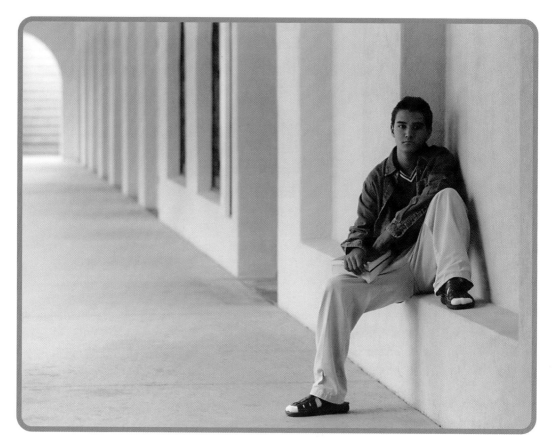

Victims of abuse often feel alone, and that they cannot confide in anyone. They may be fearful about consequences to themselves or to their abuser if they tell. What they do not realize is that the abuse is not their fault, and only by seeking help can their lives improve.

of fearfulness and anxiety, such as in PTSD, techniques that deal directly with these symptoms are extremely effective. They accomplish two results: First, they retrain the individual to be able to approach situations that frighten him without fear, which is done in a gradual and supportive manner and is called **desensitization**. Second, they help the victim correct unrealistic fears and false perceptions of their environments. This is called

cognitive restructuring. Psychotherapy is also effective with depression when it teaches specific coping behaviors and skills and corrects unrealistic ideas about oneself, other people, and the environment. When there is aggression and other behavior problems, psychotherapy is best when it involves the family and teaches effective problem solving. Most therapists believe that brief therapy may also be helpful to abused children even if they are not showing symptoms immediately after the trauma. This is done to evaluate risk of later problems and to prevent the development of unrealistic fears.

In addition to formal counseling, you may be interested in participating in support groups that exist in your community for victims of rape or abuse. In these groups you will learn that others have been going through the same pain that you feel. It is helpful to learn how others have coped, and to reach out to help them as they, in turn, extend themselves to you.

In the final analysis you must help yourself. You must learn to identify your negative thoughts, to catch yourself engaging in these thoughts, and to apply the breaks. Learn to say "STOP!" to yourself and to substitute more constructive thoughts. Review your achievements and accomplishments. Focus on your positive characteristics. Tell yourself that you are a good person. Build new skills. Make realistic plans for your future, and set goals and time frames in which to achieve these goals. Again, a counselor or your parents can help with these plans. You are not defined by your trauma.

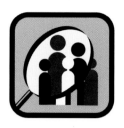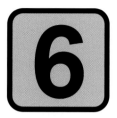

What More
Can Be Done?

Ali's father and mother were brother and sister. By age 12, he had already compiled a thick social welfare file—one that was destined to grow thicker. Ali was removed from his natural parents at a very young age, and he became a ward of the city's Child Welfare agency. He is kept unaware of his parents where-abouts—his mother is a drug user who lives on the streets, and his father is in prison for sexually molesting his children. Ali spent time in a foster home unit but that placement eventually failed as he became increasingly aggressive, inappropriate, and bizarre. A disturbed African American adolescent is not easily placed in foster homes. Now the agency feels that Ali needs the structure and safety of a psychiatric hospital. Ali is uncertain about his sexual identity and sometimes tries to dress up in woman's clothing. Other children label him as gay; Ali is not yet sure what he is.

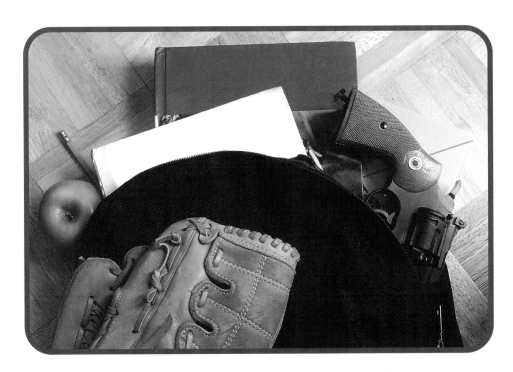

Violence by children and aimed at children seems to be a prevalent part of our society right now. Children should not have to deal with this kind of trauma, and it can often force them to grow up more quickly.

Just a few more words are needed to complete the message of this book—words that go beyond the pain of any one person or group. We need to put an end to abuse, rape, incest, and violence. As this book was being written, this country suffered the most serious attack in its history. Today's teens are not old enough to have experienced wars and there has never been an attack of such magnitude within the borders of the United States. Its impact on children has not yet been estimated, but it will undoubtedly be devastating. We need to protect children from trauma no matter what the cost. If you have been a victim, we hope this book will help you cope. We have tried to educate you about the seriousness of the problem, to make you an informed adolescent and wiser adult. We have explained why such horrors occur and have outlined the emotional havoc they produce. We have tried to familiarize you with your rights as children and have encouraged you to seek help, to reveal, to regain control, to find reason for optimism, and to move on. But we must do more than that. It is important to expand these efforts to confront the general problem, to change our country so that trauma does not happen. What can one person accomplish?

Teens who have suffered trauma grow up more quickly. You are forced to face emotional pain when your attention should be focused on school, friends, and fun. It can dampen your spirits about yourself, destroy your confidence in family and adults, and sour you about the world in which you live. That does not need to happen. In addition to the healing you must engage in to confront the challenges of adulthood, you must also be an agent of change, influencing others in a positive way. As an adult in transition, you need to learn to be sensitive to the pain of others, to extend a helping hand to those who have been traumatized, to support efforts of schools and advocates for children, and to promote legislation, education, and research.

> **How would it feel**
>
> **to deal with the emotions created by abuse while still trying to live a normal life?**

It is important that you recognize the many influences around you that promote violence. Be critical when you watch TV and see the use of weapons and force accepted as normal and desirable. Even cartoons often depict one character inflicting harm on another, as if there were no consequences. If there are guns in your home you should avoid them, except when there is responsible adult supervision. Conflicts, disagreements, and differences in opinion are a natural part of life. Solving them by the use of force is not natural. Learn ways of negotiating, compromising, and problem solving. Be sensitive to the feelings of others. Adolescence is a time of raging hormones and sexual awareness. Be wary of those who joke about rape or

What would you do

if you found your dad's gun under your parents' bed?

exploitation of others. Intimate relationships are a serious matter that involve a degree of commitment as well as mutual consent. It is not something that is imposed by force, and you should never be coerced into doing anything you don't want to sexually. When it is committed by an adult on a child it is abuse. It is illegal and should result in serious punishment for the one inflicting the abuse. But if no one knows, then the crime goes unpunished and the perpetrator is free to continue inflicting abuse.

This is the end of a book written to help you cope with the terrible things that may have happened to you. It is hoped that it will also be the beginning of a wiser, stronger, healthier you. It does not have all the answers. Abuse, rape, incest, and violence can occur anywhere. When society learns to deal with these terrible problems, the incidence of trauma to children will also be reduced. For now you must deal with your situation, your feelings. A writer once pointed out that bad things happen to good people. No one deserves to be victimized. But no matter how badly you have been treated, it is not the events alone that determine your fate but your reactions to them. Two people may process the same information in completely different ways. One will dwell on the past, brood over what happened, and color the world as a dark, threatening, dangerous place. The other will see

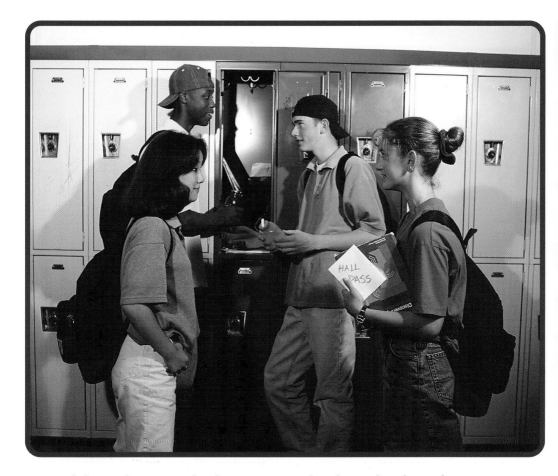

It is not the events that happen to you that determine the path you take in life, but how you react to them. If you react to a painful experience in a positive, constructive way, renewed self-confidence and learning could result. Teens who have experienced violence or abuse can use their experiences to educate others, and to spread a message of prevention to their contemporaries.

the trauma as a terrible thing that happened in the past, but place it in perspective of new options and opportunities. Let today be the beginning of a happier, more competent, more optimistic you. Let it also be the beginning of your efforts to change America, one person at a time.

Glossary

Acquaintance/date rape – a rape committed by someone the victim knows or has dated; the most common form of rape committed against girls aged 15-25.

Aggression – hostile, injurious, or destructive behavior or outlook caused by frustration.

Attachment – the bonding that takes place between an infant and his or her mother and father.

Attachment disorder – some disruption of the normal attachment process, the presence of which psychologists have found is a significant predictor of abuse children.

Battered child syndrome – serious physical injury inflicted on a child that cannot be explained by medical history, and must by law be reported to the authorities.

Civil rights movement – activism that began in the 1950s and seeks full human rights for oppressed groups such as minorities, the handicapped, and children.

Cognitive restructuring – a technique through which a therapist helps a patient correct his or her unrealistic fears and false perceptions about the environment.

Conduct disorder – when an impulse control disorder becomes so severe that it violates the rights of others.

Convention on the Human Rights of the Child – a policy adopted by UNICEF in 1989 that affirms fundamental human dignity, the family's role in the life of the child, and children's right for respect.

Culture of violence – the overwhelming presence of violence and violent images in neighborhoods, families, and on TV and in movies that makes a person less likely to empathize with the pain and suffering of others.

Glossary

Desensitization – a technique used by a therapist to retrain a patient to approach situations that frighten him or her without fear.

Flashbacks – a vivid reliving of a past traumatic experience that appears real to the individual experiencing it.

Incest – any sexual activity between blood relatives, whether or not it is consensual.

Impulse control – the ability to control one's desires.

Impulse control disorder – a psychiatric condition that describes people who cannot manage their anger when they are thwarted in their desires.

Neglect – the failure to provide adequate medical attention, nutrition, or protection from exposure to the elements.

Privileged communication law – the law that ensures that everything you say to a therapist remains private, except when it has to do with child abuse.

Post-traumatic stress disorder (PTSD) – an anxiety disorder in which prior traumatic experiences such as abuse are recalled only in flashbacks, nightmares, night terrors, and other psychiatric symptoms.

Racism – discrimination against a particular group solely on the basis of characteristics such as ethnicity, religion, age, or gender.

Rape – forced sexual intercourse with a person, when sex is not desired or solicited in any way.

Trauma – a disordered psychological or behavioral state resulting from mental or emotional stress or physical injury.

Victimization – to make someone a victim through acts like rape, incest, and violence.

Violence – physical trauma inflicted on one person by another.

Further Reading

Books:

Ackerman, R.J. and Graham, D. *Too Old to Cry: Abused Teens in Today's America.* New York: McGraw-Hill, 1990.

Harill, S.E. *Empowering Teens to Build Self-esteem.* Houston: Innerworks, 1999.

Hersch, P. *A Tribe Apart: A Journey into the Heart of American Adolescence.* New York: Ballantine, 1998.

Hipp, E. and Hanson, L.K. *Understanding the Human Volcano: What Teens Can Do About Violence.* Center City, MN: Hazelden Information & Educational Services, 2000.

Sayers, J. *Boy Crazy: Remembering Adolescence, Therapies, and Dreams.* New York: Routledge, 1993.

Ward, F., Ward, B., and Olszewski, L.J. *About Sexual Abuse: A program for teens and young adults.* Boston: Unitarian Universalist Association, 1999.

Websites:

www.rainn.org

www.kidshealth.org

www.childabuse.org

www.ncpc.org

Index

Index

About the Author

Marvin Rosen is a licensed clinical psychologist who practices in Media, Pennsylvania. He received his doctorate degree from the University of Pennsylvania in 1961. Since 1963, he has worked with intellectually and emotionally challenged people at Elwyn, Inc. in Pennsylvania, with clinical, administrative, research, and training responsibilities. He also conducts a private practice of psychology. Dr. Rosen has taught psychology at the University of Pennsylvania, Bryn Mawr College, and West Chester University. He has written or edited seven book and numerous professional articles in the areas of psychology, rehabilitation, emotional disturbance, and mental retardation.